101 Uses of Essential Oils

A Safe Guide To Aromatherapy In Everyday Life

by Ann Sullivan

Published in USA by:

Ann Sullivan
217 N. Seacrest Blvd #9
Boynton Beach
FL 33425

© Copyright 2015

ISBN-13: ISBN-13: 978-1544738130
ISBN-10: ISBN-10: 1544738137

Table of Contents

Introduction

When you hear or read about essential oils, you're often told how beneficial and versatile these natural oils can be. Though these claims are true, you – the intelligent consumer – would probably like more substantial evidence to back them rather than just the same old taglines. Knowing the basic components of essential oils will lay the groundwork for a better understanding of why these natural oils are, in fact, so essential when it comes to your home, your wellness, and your body.

First things first – it's important to understand that essential oils are not oils in the normal sense of the word, because they are not composed of the fatty acids that you find in olive oil, sunflower oil, or other cooking oils. Instead, it is made up of highly concentrated plant constituents that promote medicinal qualities, and various other qualities, which make them suitable for household cleaning, therapeutic uses, cosmetic uses, and many other valuable uses that we will discuss in this book.

The reason that essential oils are so vital for medicinal and household cleaning purposes is that they possess antiviral, antifungal, and antibacterial properties. Those oils that are particularly valuable in this way are lemon, eucalyptus, melaleuca, grapefruit, peppermint, rosemary and lavender.

When it comes to cosmetics and personal care products, essential oils are applicable because of the easy absorption through the skin due to the oil's tiny molecular size. Because of this keen ability to absorb and evaporate, the healing, nourishing, and softening properties of essential oils allow the molecules to do their job and then leave the skin, rather than accumulating over time.

Perhaps essential oils are best known for their therapeutic and aromatic properties. Lavender and rosemary oils, for instance, help relax the body; and, further, rosemary has been shown to boost brain performance, particularly in recounting information for exams. However, know that "fragrance oil" or "perfume" is not the same as essential oil. These pretenders are not natural, but synthetic, and so do not carry any of the benefits that essential oils do.

Essential oils are entirely natural, so they cannot be patented or used in pharmaceuticals. This is why you will not find the average healthcare practitioner prescribing natural essential oils instead of synthetic drugs. The fact that the oils cannot be patented steers drug companies away from them altogether, as they see no money in the organic oil. Moreover, the mainstream makes no efforts to study the oils, so available research is often based on experimentation garnered over centuries, or for as long as essential oils have been in use.

What we do know, from so many years of practical knowledge, is that essential oils are extremely concentrated, which is what makes them so powerful...and possibly potent if used incorrectly. For instance, before using topically, almost all essential oils should be diluted with carrier oils (those fatty acid oils we talked about), or alcohols, waxes, butters, or any other dilutions suggested. Without diluting these highly concentrated oils, your skin will, at best, not receive them well; at worst, undiluted essential oils may create a terrible allergic reaction.

To illustrate why these oils are so concentrated, in extreme cases, a single pound of rose oil is produced by 4000 pounds of Bulgarian roses, while in less extreme cases – like lavender's, for instance – a single pound of oil is produced by 100 pounds of the plant. Either way, it's obvious that the concentration of these plant components is incredibly high, giving them the potential to harm if used incorrectly.

Simply put, know the oils you are using. Some are safe to use undiluted – like melaleuca, lavender, German chamomile, and sandalwood –, while it's necessary to combine others with carrier oils. It's also important to know your patient. Children, pregnant women, and the elderly require different remedies, and in most cases, further dilution. A baby, or child, has thinner skin than do adults, so always use diluted essential oils when treating them, and only half of the dosage recommended. Pregnant women, or those who are nursing, should not be treated with clove, cinnamon, cedarwood, rosemary, lemon, ginger, clary sage, chamomile. If you are unsure about treating a patient in certain conditions with an oil, always check with your practitioner.

If you're not sure whether you or your patient will be sensitive to a particular oil, test it on the upper portion of the arm, combining ½ tsp carrier oil (fractionated coconut oil) with one drop of essential oil. Rub the mixture into your skin and allow to sit for several hours. Unless your skin starts to itch, or there's a reaction on the skin's surface, you may consider the oil safe for use.

Other safety precautions include avoiding contact between essential oils and your eyes, steering clear of those essential oils for which you may have an allergy, and keeping the oils out of reach of children, as you would with any medication. Though essential oils are natural, the high concentration means they can be harmful, or even toxic (though this is uncommon), when undiluted. In fact, you should never ingest essential oils unless highly diluted. Essential oils are most commonly used topically or aromatically.

When purchasing essential oils, you should also consider the brand and the oil quality. High cost does not always equate to better quality. In fact, you can test the quality of essential oils by placing a drop onto a strip of construction paper. The quicker it evaporates without leaving a ring, the purer it is. If it does leave a ring, the manufacturer has diluted the product with another oil.

Some brands that aren't as expensive are perfectly acceptable for cleaning, or for other non-therapeutic uses. It's also safe to go with the cheaper of those more expensive and better quality brands that vary only slightly in price, as they likely come from the same source. There are only a few essential oil distilleries throughout the world, so the quality between these products differs little.

One bottle of essential oil can last you 5 to 10 years when stored correctly (apart from citrus oils, which only last a couple of years at most), so though a small bottle may seem expensive, the longevity of its life expectancy makes it a cost-effective purchase. This is due to the high concentration of the oils – often, only a drop or two is required. When storing, keep the product out of direct sunlight in the dark glass bottles they were packaged in, so that they remain effective.

This basic introduction to essential oils has hopefully clarified the components of essential oils and provided answers as to why these natural agents of the earth are so beneficial. In this book, we will take a look at the many uses of essential oils, from the home to your wellness, from the aromatic to the therapeutic, and from cosmetic to practical. The applications of essential oils are unending, so you will be sure to find a number of uses specific to you.

Chapter 1:
Essential Oils for Aroma

It is commonly known that the sense of smell is the strongest of the 5 senses in relation to memory. When a person smells a certain aroma, or a certain scent, they can easily recall a memory from their past corresponding with this same aroma or scent. This is because the olfactory bulb, which is connected to the sense of smell, is actually a working part of the limbic system of our brains, linked to feelings, memories, and emotions. When scents are associated with memories, they produce instant recollections and extreme responses. Scents can also affect a person's mood and work performance.

The brain's hippocampus is involved in associative learning, and the amygdala processes emotion. Since the olfactory bulb is connected to both, memories can be triggered through conditioned reactions, such as those occurring when you initially smelled a particular scent that was linked to a particular person, place, thing, or event. For instance, the smell of a rose may be linked to a rose garden from your youth, or the smell of chlorine may link to those summers spent at the local pool. The next time you come into contact with this same scent, a mood or memory will be stimulated by that preexisting link. For this reason, everyone's favorite scents differ, as they are each linked to different people, places, things, or events.

This is why using essential oils for aromatic purposes can alter a person's mood – because the sense of smell is so strongly linked to memory and mood, and you can choose those which recall the best memories. Below are several ways to use oils aromatically.

#1 Oil Burner

This is perhaps the most common way to use essential oils for aromatic purposes. When using essential oils in an oil burner, choose your scent and, with an eyedropper, distribute 5-10 drops of your chosen oil into the burner's bowl, along with several drops of purified water. Put a tea light below the bowl, and the scent will quickly waft throughout the room.

#2 Diffuser

Another easier and safer method for burning oils for aromatic purposes is with a diffuser. Diffusers don't require a flame. You simply distribute several drops in the diffuser's bowl and plug the diffuser in. Diffusers are great to create a stimulating scent in the home or office. Choose whichever aroma pleases you.

#3 Furnace Filter

By placing a couple drops of essential oil on a furnace filter, the scent will spread throughout your house once you turn on the furnace fan. Cinnamon bark, vanilla, cypress, cassia, or pine are all fantastic holiday scents...particularly, if you have a fake Christmas tree.

#4 Air Purifier

To clarify, this will purify the scent in the air, not the air itself. For example, if you want to rid the air of cigarette smoke, you can use a combination of melaleuca, rosemary, and eucalyptus. Place a 1/4 cup of water and 4 drops of each oil into a spray bottle and shake vigorously before each use. To distribute in the air, simply spray in a circular motion.

#5 Paint Fume Dilution

If you have a big paint project in your home, you can dilute the paint fumes by combining 10 milliliters of peppermint oil with a gallon of paint. This will reduce the unpleasant fumes.

#6 Deodorizer

Those with stinky feet may benefit from applying a couple drops of lemon, or geranium oil, either directly in the shoes, or onto a cotton ball left inside the shoes overnight. This will get rid of the odor in the shoes and provide your feet a fresh scent once the shoes are removed.

#7 Car Diffuser

Instead of hanging the usual old evergreen tree from your rearview mirror, use a car diffuser to keep your car smelling fresher, longer. Apply 2-8 drops of your favorite essential oil onto the diffuser's pad and insert it into the diffuser. If you have a tendency towards road rage, use lavender, vanilla, rosemary, or lemon as all are known to relieve stress.

#8 Studying Stimulant

As we discussed in the introduction to aromatic uses of essential oils, scents stimulate memories. The power of aroma concentrated in essential oils means that they are even stronger memory stimulants than your average scent. They also boost alertness and concentration, great for studying, or for writing that last-minute research paper. Peppermint and grapefruit are particularly nice for driving, as they promote alertness, while bergamot and basil increase your concentration. Several different essential oils can be used as inhalants to stimulate focus.

#9 Air Freshener

For a basic air freshener, simply mix 10-20 drops of your favorite oil with 16 ounces of purified water. Pour these in a spray bottle and shake thoroughly before each use. The great thing about using essential oils is that you can personalize your own blend with your favorite scents. Also, as you can make these blends on-the-spot, the air freshener will always be strong and long-lasting.

#10 Peace-Maker

If things have been tense, either in your home or at work, and you're looking to promote a peaceful environment, grapefruit and lavender both relieve stress and induce feelings of relaxation and peace. You can use with an oil burner, diffused, or as an air freshener.

#11 Fresh Linen

Have you ever been a guest in someone's home and their bed linen or towels smell out of this world? Well, yours can too, when you apply 10-15 drops of essential oil to a square of terry cloth and use as a dryer sheet. For the same result, you can also mix 5 drops of oil with a 1/4 cup water and pour it into your washer's center cup along with your clothes, sheets, and towels. Your linen will come out smelling of rose, lavender, geranium, or whatever scent you wish. Also, if you've recently had insect infestation in your linens, like bed mites, eucalyptus essential oil will help eliminate them.

#12 The Great Outdoors

During the winter holidays, many folks want their homes to smell like the strong scent of Christmas, as it recalls their childhood. You can produce a penetrating holiday aroma throughout your home by scenting your firewood. Using sage, frankincense, myrrh, or pine, and apply 8-10 drops of the selected oil to a dry log. Let sit for a time before burning, as the oil must soak in for the best effect. For your safety, never put oil on an already lit fire.

#13 Stationary Scent

You can scent most anything with essential oils, but continuing with the holiday theme, you might consider scenting your annual Christmas card to set it apart from the rest. Fir needle, cassia, or cinnamon are excellent holiday scents. In fact, you can scent all your outgoing cards at once by placing your cards in a sealable plastic bag, along with a few drops of your selected oil applied to a piece of paper. Seal the bag and allow the stationary to soak in the scent overnight. You can do this with any paper products, but be careful, as the oil may leave marks if in contact with the paper or cards being scented.

#14 Candle Scent

Whether you make your own candles or buy unscented ones, you can add your own scent by applying several drops of your selected oil to the melting wax. 3 drops of vanilla, orange, or whichever scent you choose will do. You can also make insect-repelling candles using lemon, eucalyptus, or citronella oils. Just be sure to add the oil when the candle is unlit.

Chapter 2:
Essential Oils for the Home

Kitchen

#15 Floor Wipes

DIY Floor Wipes

Ingredients:

- 1 ½ cups water*
- (*distilled for long-term use; tap for short-term use)
- ½ cup rubbing alcohol
- 1 ½ cups white vinegar

- 5 drops melaleuca, 5 drops peppermint, 10 drops orange
- Materials
- Swiffer
- 4-6 washcloths

Instructions:

Step 1: Roll 4-6 washcloths and stuff them into a jar.

Step 2: Stir together vinegar, water, essential oils, and rubbing alcohol in a small bowl.

Step 3: Pour this blend into the jar until the washcloths are fully immersed. If your washcloths are bigger, add more vinegar and water. Press the cloths into the liquid then shut the jar's lid.

Step 4: As needed, take a washcloth from the jar and attach it to a Swiffer mop. Mop the floor, as usual. When finished, throw the washcloth into the washer and use again, repeating the process.

Note: When attaching the washcloth to the Swiffer, secure the cloths ends in the slots on the base's top. Reverse the cloth half-way through cleaning for the best results.

#16 Trash Deodorizer

When your trashcan starts to produce that awful lingering smell, place a few drops of any essential oil onto a cotton ball and put in the bottom of the can, beneath the trash bag. This is also a good solution for diaper pails. Not only does the oil reduce the odor, but it will kill germs.

#17 Stovetop Cleaner

DIY Stovetop Cleaner

Ingredients

- 5 ounces distilled water
- 5 ounces white vinegar
- 1 teaspoon baking soda
- 20 drops lemon oil

Instructions

Step 1: Combine vinegar and water in a large bowl.

Step 2: Gradually add the baking soda. The combination will likely fizz, so be careful!

Step 3: Stir in the lemon oil.

Step 4: Pour into an 11-ounce glass spray bottle, spray down the stovetop and scrub.

#18 Fruit Preserver

Tired of your fruit going bad before you even get a chance to eat it? This recipe will both clean your fruit and lengthen its shelf life. Apply 2-6 drops of lemon essential oil to a bowl of cool water. Wash the fruit before setting it into the fruit keeper. Place the fruit in the basin and stir. Dry and return to fruit dish for longer-lasting fruit.

#19 Cooking Deodorizer

Your daughter accidently left dinner on the stove too long and the whole kitchen smells of burnt chicken, a scent that will linger for years...or until you throw together this cooking deodorizer. Combine purified water and cinnamon, clove, or citrus essential oil in a pan. Let simmer for 10-15 minutes, or until the odor has dissipated.

#20 Appliance Cleanser

When you're preparing the final rinse water to clean kitchen appliances – like your oven, refrigerator or freezer, for instance – add several drops of lemongrass, lime, grapefruit, or bergamot to your washrag for a lasting sparkle and an especially fresh scent.

#21 Liquid Dish Soap

DIY Liquid Dish Soap

Ingredients

- 1 ½ cups water
- ¼ cup tightly packed grated Dr. Bronner's bar soap
- ¼ cup liquid castile soap
- ½ teaspoon non-GMO glycerin
- 1 tablespoon super washing soda*
- (*adjust by up to 1 teaspoon for desired thickness)
- 15-40 drops essential oil*
- (*lemon, lime, and orange help cut grease)

Instructions

Step 1: In a large saucepan, heat the water on the stove over medium-high. Then grate the Dr. Bronner's soap into the water, stirring until it dissolves.

Step 2: Remove the soapy mixture from heat and transfer to container (preferably the pump dispenser, if the mouth is wide enough).

Step 3: Mix in glycerin, washing soda, and liquid castile soap and stir.

Step 4: Stirring occasionally, allow to sit for 24 hours,

and then check the thickness. Runny liquid soap is fine, as the product will thicken as it ages. However, if you'd prefer thicker soap, reheat it and dissolve ¾ teaspoon washing soda into the soap, allowing it to sit for 24 hours again. Repeat until you've reached the desired consistency.

Step 5: If you haven't already, add the soap to a dispenser.

Note:

If there are clumps in your soap, then blend or mix in the blender. Also, the soap will thicken over time. When it does, simply mix in some warm or hot water and shake your dispenser well.

#22 Kitchen Sink Scrub

If your sink has become grimy or you simply wish to disinfect it, combine 1/8 cup vinegar, ½ cup baking soda, 5 drops of lime oil and 5 drops of bergamot oil. Scrub this mixture into the sink and wash down with warm water for a sparkling finish.

#23 Grease Cutter

With a three-ingredient grease-fighting formula of ¼ cup castile soap, 2 cups water and 10 drops lavender oil, you can eliminate grease quickly on your stove, countertops, sink, or dishes.

#24 Dishwasher Additive

Prior to the wash cycle, add 2 drops of lemon oil into your dishwashing detergent. Not only will it give your dishes an added sparkle, it will deodorize your dishwasher in an eco-friendly way.

Living Room

#25 Wood Polish

DIY Wood Polish

Ingredients

- ¾ cup water
- 2 tablespoons vodka*
- (*may replace with white vinegar)
- 1 tablespoon olive oil
- 2 tablespoons white vinegar
- 1 tablespoon liquid glycerin (optional)
- 30-40 drops essential oil (lemon, orange, clove)
- ½ teaspoon melted emulsifying wax
- ¼ teaspoon xanthan gum

Instructions

Step 1: Mix together olive oil, water, vinegar, vodka,

glycerin, and essential oil in a blender on high.

Step 2: Add the emulsifying wax and the xanthan gum while continuing to blend for 10-15 seconds. The mixture should be somewhat thick.

Step 3: Pour the mixture into a spritz bottle, and apply on wooden surfaces as usual.

Note: Product expires in around 3 months.

#26 Carpet Deodorizer

You've just moved into a new home or apartment, and the last resident left an odor that's been absorbed into the carpet. Never fear – this strong and natural carpet deodorizer will eliminate the odor and leave your home smelling fresh. Combine a box of baking soda with 5-10 drops of peppermint, lavender, lemon, geranium, ylang ylang, or any essential oil of your choice and mix thoroughly. Sprinkle the mixture over your carpets and allow to rest for an hour or longer. The baking soda will absorb the stench and the oil will leave its refreshing scent. Vacuum the mixture up, and your home's air is as good as new.

#27 Vacuum Scent

If your household has a dog, then chances are, no matter how clean you keep him, your carpet and home will carry the dog's odor. You can help eliminate this odor every time you vacuum by applying 5 drops of whichever essential oil you choose to a cotton ball. Geranium is best to rid of animal scents, while pine, peppermint, cassia, or spearmint will leave your home smelling fresh. Put the cotton ball in your vacuum cleaner bag, and the pleasant scent will be emitted whenever you clean.

#28 Leather Cleaner

DIY Leather Cleaner

Ingredients

- ¼ cup olive oil
- ¼ cup vinegar
- 10 drops lemon or orange essential oil

Instructions

Step 1: Vacuum your furniture to remove it of debris and dust. Wipe down with a damp paper towel.

Step 2: Combine olive oil and vinegar in a container and mix well (the two won't mix entirely).

Step 3: Stir in essential oil.

Step 4: Dampen a paper towel with the cleaner. To test it, rub the cleaner gently into a small section of leather and allow to dry for 20 minutes before checking for discoloration. If there is none, coat the furniture completely, rubbing the cleaner in a circular motion.

Step 5: Using a dry paper towel, wipe the furniture down to remove any oil residue.

Bathroom

#29 Toilet Bombs

DIY Toilet Bombs

Ingredients

- ½ cup citric acid (from lemons or oranges)
- 1 1/3 cup baking soda
- 30 drops lemon essential oil
- 30 drops lavender essential oil
- 30 drops peppermint essential oil

Instructions

Step 1: Combine the citric acid and baking soda.

Step 2: Combine the oils in a spray bottle and spray bit by bit into the mixture, stirring continuously.

Step 3: Add a little water if mixture isn't moist enough – but not too much, otherwise the bombs won't fizz.

Step 4: Using a muffin pan or silicone mold, divide the mixture amongst the dishes and allow to set for six hours.

Step 5: Store the bombs in an airtight container, and drop one into the toilet bowl to clean. The bomb will fizz, killing the bacteria, cleaning, and deodorizing.

#30 Bathroom Deodorizer

Do you want a bathroom that doesn't smell like one? Another very simple bathroom deodorizer involves a cotton ball and a few drops of essential oil. Place 3 drops of lemon, lavender, or lime on a cotton ball and set behind the toilet, or under the sink to keep your bathroom smelling fresh.

#31 Bathroom Tile, Sink, and Bath Cleaner

To clean your bathroom's sink, bath, and tiles, combine ½ cup castile soap, 2/3 cup baking soda, ½ cup water, 2 tablespoons vinegar and 3-5 drops of melaleuca oil in a squirt bottle. Shake thoroughly. The mixture will be thick and pasty, which is why it's ideal to clean the buildup and mildew frequently found in bathrooms.

#32 Bathroom Sanitizer

Lemon essential oil is a simple, easy-to-use bathroom

sanitizer. Apply several drops to a paper towel and wipe down all bathroom fixtures to kill bacteria and give your bathroom a fresh scent and streak-free shine.

Laundry Room

#33 Laundry Detergent

Buy unscented laundry detergent or make your own (see recipe below). If you choose to buy unscented detergent, simply add 3-5 drops of lavender, frankincense, or a citrus oil to the single-portion of detergent prior to each load.

DIY Laundry Detergent

Ingredients

- 1 box of washing soda
- 1 bar of unscented castile soap
- 1 box of borax
- 4 ½ gallons of water

Directions

Step 1: Using a food processor or a cheese grater, grate the castile soap into a fine powder with no lumps.

Step 2: Dissolve the soap flakes by heating them with 2 quarts of water in a saucepan over medium heat, stirring continuously until dissolved.

Step 3: Using tap water, heat 4 ½ gallons in a large pot until the water is nearly boiling. When it's ready, pour the water into a 5-gallon bucket, and add 1 cup of borax and 1 cup of washing soda. Stir until dissolved.

Step 4: Add the soapy water to the mix, and stir well.

Step 5: Cover and allow to rest overnight.

Step 6: Distribute into sealable storage containers.

Step 7: For best results, add your chosen essential oil to each single-measurement. Large loads use 1 cup of the detergent and 3-6 drops of oil. Small loads use ½ cup of detergent and 1-3 drops of oil.

Recommended Oil Blends

Floral blends: 2-parts lavender to 1-part rosemary, or 2-parts lavender to 1-part vanilla, or equal parts wild orange and geranium

Sultry blends: equal parts geranium and rose, or 2-parts lemon to 1-part chamomile to 1-part lemongrass

Citrus blends: equal parts wild orange and lemon, or equal parts melaleuca, lemon and lemongrass

#34 Dryer Sheets

These eco-friendly dryer sheets are also cost-effective and reusable. With no toxic additives and your favorite scent, your clothes will be soft and smelling fresh. Vinegar naturally softens your clothing, while the oil cleans and provides a fresh scent. Simply combine ½ cup vinegar and 8 drops of melaleuca oil, or your favorite scent. Using dollar store dish towels, old linen or t-shirts, cut your cotton cloths down to small squares, and pour the mixture over the cloths to dampen them. Store in an airtight container until needed, then take one sheet, squeeze the excess liquid into the container, and add to your dryer load. Once used, replace the sheet in the jar for future use.

#35 Linen Spray

DIY Linen Spray

Ingredients

2 tablespoons pure grain alcohol (everclear or vodka)

2 cups distilled water

12-18 drops essential oil or blend

Instructions

Step 1: Combine alcohol with essential oil in a glass container. The oils must dissolve in the alcohol, so let sit for 15-30 minutes.

Step 2: Combine alcohol-oil mixture with distilled water and mix well.

Step 3: Pour the mixture into spray bottles.

Step 4: Shake before each use. Spray linens, curtains, or other fabrics with 1-3 sprays. Do not use as a perfume.

#36 Fabric Softener

To make your own fabric softener, you'll need 1 cup baking soda, 1 cup distilled water, 2 cups white vinegar and 25 drops of lavender oil. Whisk together the oil and the baking soda in a large bowl then gradually pour in the vinegar. The mixture will begin to fizz. Once it's done, transfer the fabric softener into an airtight container and use as normal. Shake well before each use.

#37 Bleach for Laundry

Laundry bleach can be made by combining ½ cup hydrogen peroxide (3% solution), 3 ¼ cups water, 5 drops lemon essential oil, and 2 tablespoons lemon juice or ½ teaspoon citric acid. This recipe makes one quart of bleach. Use one cup per load of laundry.

Other

#38 Deodorizing Disks

DIY Deodorizing Disks

Ingredients

- 1-2 cups distilled water*
- (*alternatively, you can boil water for 10 minutes and allow to cool)
- 2 cups baking soda
- 2-4 drops lavender or citrus essential oil

Instructions

Step 1: Combine ½ cup distilled water with 3-4 drops

essential oil.

Step 2: Add mixture to 2 cups baking soda and mix thoroughly.

Step 3: Your mixture should be the consistency of a thick paste. Add water until it reaches that point.

Step 4: Using a muffin pan or silicone mold, divide the mixture into separate cups to create your deodorizing disks.

Step 5: Allow 24-48 hours to dry and harden.

Step 6: Use in smelly trash cans, diaper bins, or compactors for up to a month. You can even add the used disk to a load of laundry when the potency fades to give your clothing or linen some added scent.

#39 All-Purpose Cleaner

To create a great all-purpose cleaner with antimicrobial properties, combine 2 teaspoons of melaleuca oil with 2 cups of water in a spray bottle and shake thoroughly before each use.

#40 General Cleaner

Another cleaner for general use on countertops, mirrors, or other surfaces, combine 20 drops of lemon or lemongrass essential oil, ½ cup water, and ½ cup apple cider vinegar or white vinegar. These oils have strong antimicrobial properties, which kill e.Coli and salmonella.

#41 Disinfectant

For an effective disinfectant, fill a bowl with water and several drops of lemon essential oil. Put a dishcloth in the bowl and allow to soak overnight. The disinfectant will kill germs, so the cloth can be used to wipe down countertops, tables or any surfaces.

#42 Dish, Counter & Floor Cleaner

Fill a bucket or sink with 1 ½ gallons of hot water, along with 5-10 drops of spearmint, lemon or melaleuca oil, and a capful of unscented dish soap. This combination can be used to wash dishes, mop the floor, or clean countertops.

#43 Mold Killer

To kill unhealthy mold in your home, combine 10 drops of lavender oil with ½ cup distilled white vinegar in a spray bottle and shake thoroughly. An alternative recipe combines 2 cups of water with 2 teaspoons melaleuca oil. With either option, spray the mixture on the mold and let sit. Do not wash or rinse the spray off.

#44 Moth Repellant

Moths and clothes do not mix. You can repel these

destructive insects by applying several drops of patchouli oil to a cotton ball and placing it strategically in each closet of your home.

#45 Fly Repellant

Shooing flies never seems to do the job. To get rid of them, combine 16 ounces of purified water with 25 drops of lavender or peppermint oil in a spray bottle. Shake thoroughly before using, and spray any potential entryways where flies might be able to enter the home. Also spray counter tops and windows to deter them from landing on your home's surfaces, inside and out.

#46 Mice Repellant

Mice infestations make for an unsanitary home environment. To get rid of the little diseased rodents, combine 1 cup of water with 2 teaspoons of peppermint essential oil in a spray bottle. Shake well and spray those areas frequented by mice or those where you've seen mouse damage. You can also leave a cotton ball soaked in 3-6 drops of peppermint at entryways. This oil also deters squirrels, spiders, and other insects and rodents.

#47 Soft-Scrubber

DIY 4-Way Soft-Scrubber

Ingredients

- 1 ½ cups baking soda*
- (*you may use less or more as needed)
- 10 drops lavender, melaleuca, or rosemary essential oil
- ½ cup liquid laundry detergent or soap

Instructions

Step 1: In a bowl, mix ½ cup baking soda with ½ cup laundry detergent. Add more and more baking soda and teaspoons of water until the combination reaches a cake frosting consistency.

Step 2: Add essential oil.

Step 3: Put this mixture into an airtight container.

Step 4: Use the soft scrub with a damp rag to clean faucets or sinks, toilets, stainless steel, pots and pans, silver, coffee stains, tile grout, countertops, stovetops, and much more.

Note: Add water if the mixture starts to dry.

#48 Adhesive Remover

When you find gum, glue, crayon, oil or other adhesives stuck to the floor, wall or other surfaces, try removing it with a rag soaked in 1-2 drops of lemon essential oil. The lemon oil aids in the removal of adhesives.

#49 Cleaning Bleach

Cleaning with bleach rids of household mold, bacteria and viruses, because of its potency. You can make your own quart-size cleaning bleach with this simple recipe: 2 cups water, 2 cups hydrogen peroxide (3% solution), 10 drops lemon essential oil, and ½ teaspoon citric acid or 2 tablespoons lemon juice. Pour the mixture into a spray bottle. Light exposure weakens the mixture, so if you want it to last longer than a month, you must store it in the dark, or in covered containers. For simple and quick storage, keep the spray bottle in a brown paper bag tied at the top, and the bleach will last for up to three months.

#50 Spot Stain Remover

DIY Spot Stain Remover

Ingredients

- 2 drops eucalyptus, peppermint or lemon essential oil

- 2 tablespoons cream of tartar
- Water

Instructions

Step 1: Mix the cream of tartar and the essential oil of choice in a small cup, adding enough water to make a paste.

Step 2: Cover the stain with the paste, and allow to dry.

Step 3: Wash stain as usual with soap and water.

Note: Spot Stain Remover works on wine, ketchup, soda, coffee, or sauce spills. Can remove stains on clothes, carpets, or other fabrics. Make as needed.

Chapter 3:
Essential Oils for Body

#51 Teeth

5 Essential Oils for Teeth & Gums

Cinnamon Essential Oil

Cinnamon essential oil possesses antibacterial and antifungal properties, and is a particularly effective antimicrobial agent, attacking the bacteria that stimulates tooth decay, called streptococcus mutans, and the bacteria that promotes gum disease, called lactobacillus plantarum.

Clove Essential Oil

Used for centuries in traditional Chinese medicine, clove essential oil prevents pathogenic bacteria, aiding the relief of tooth pain. Clove's germicidal properties also make it a good disinfectant for problematic root canals.

Myrrh essential oil

Myrrh essential oil works as a pain reliever and antiseptic. Traditionally, myrrh has been used to soothe mouth ulcers and promote gum hygiene. Myrrh promotes quick healing of gum tissue after flossing or brushing.

Peppermint essential oil

The mouth is a low-oxygen environment, so anaerobic bacteria thrive there and cause gum disease. Peppermint oil, however, effectively eliminates this particular bacteria, helping in the prevention of gum disease.

Spearmint essential oil

Spearmint is a powerful antiseptic as well, killing germs and healing wounds. Like peppermint essential oil, spearmint helps prevent gum disease by soothing and healing soft gum tissue.

#52 Massage Oil

Essential oil can, of course, be used for massage therapy. Combine with a carrier oil (fractionated coconut oil), adding a few drops of ginger for lower back pain or peppermint for sore muscles. You might also try a blend of 2 drops each of bergamot, German chamomile, lavender, and ylang ylang, along with 5 teaspoons of a carrier oil for a seriously stress-relieving massage.

#53 Nail Strengthener

To strengthen nails, combine 2 tablespoons of Vitamin E oil with 10 drops each of lemon, myrrh, and frankincense essential oils. Stir thoroughly and store in a dark glass bottle, applying to your nail cuticles twice weekly.

#54 Foot Bath

Fill a large bucket with hot water, and add 5-8 drops of rosemary or peppermint essential oil. Add 2 drops of cypress oil as well, if you wish to prevent odor or perspiration. Mix well, and place your feet in the scented bath. These oils help improve circulation and provide pain relief.

#55 Pore Cleanser

If you have clogged pores, you can cleanse them with a few drops of melaleuca, lemon, or wild orange oil on a cotton ball. Rub the soaked cotton ball gently on the affected area, and your pores will breathe easier.

#56 Soothing Bath

There are a thousand-and-one combinations when it comes to bathing with essential oils. This combination is specifically designed to produce a calming and soothing result. Blend together 1 drop Roman chamomile, 5 drops lavender, and 1 drop wild orange and stir together in your bathwater to stimulate relaxation. You can also make bath salts simply by adding ¼-1 teaspoon of the essential oil of your choice to 1 cup Epsom salt, sea salt, or baking soda. Keep your bath salt sealed in an airtight container and use as needed.

#57 Anti-Aging Cream

To reduce facial wrinkles, combine 2 tablespoons carrier oil with 3 drops lavender, 5 drops sandalwood, 6 drops frankincense and 4 drops geranium. Keep in a dark jar or container and apply as needed to affected area. Avoid your eyes.

#58 Reduce Hair Loss

If your hair has started to thin, you can prevent hair loss by adding 3 drops of rosemary essential oil to a single-size portion of shampoo or conditioner. Use as normal to stimulate scalp circulation. You can also create your own hair loss blend in a small container by combining 2 ounces of Jojoba carrier oil with 3 drops each of lavender, cedarwood, and rosemary. Shake vigorously before use and massage into the scalp for 5 minutes. Allow to sit in hair for 1 hour before washing, and use the blend twice a week. You can further stimulate hair thickness and growth by applying 1-2 drops rosemary to your hair brush before using.

#59 Eliminate Dandruff

Skip the medicated shampoos and create your own dandruff-eliminating blend by combining 2 tablespoons carrier oil with 1 drop rosemary, 5 drops lemon, 2 drops lavender and 2 drops peppermint. Apply to scalp, massaging it into your hair for 1-2 minutes. Wait 10 minutes before shampooing hair as usual.

#60 Hot Oil Conditioner for Dry Hair

Transform your dry hair to a mane that's shiny, sleek and smooth, with this super soft hot oil conditioner. In a small plastic bag, combine 4 tablespoons carrier oil with 5 drops each of lavender, geranium, and sandalwood, along with 15 drops rosewood. Heat water to a boil and fill a cup with the boiling water. To heat your oils, place the bag in the cup for 1 minute. Apply in your hair from scalp to ends then wrap your hair in a towel. Let sit for 20 minutes before washing as usual.

#61 Oily Hair remedy

For those with oily hair, blend together in a small

container 2 tablespoons carrier oil with 9 drops each of rosemary, lime, and ylang ylang. Shake well and massage into your head, starting from the scalp to the ends of your hair. Let sit for a couple minutes and then wash hair as usual. Apply this blend twice a week.

#62 Skin Toner

To create a soft and effective skin toner, combine in a bottle 2 drops each of rosewood, lavender, and geranium and 8 ounces of purified water. Cap the bottle and shake well. To apply, soak a cotton ball in the toner and rub gently on your skin. Allow the mixture to air dry. Shake bottle before each use and apply as needed.

#64 Reduce Stretch Marks

This salve is a safe, chemical-free method for pregnant women to prevent or reduce stretch marks. Combine 5 drops of carrier oil with 5 drops myrrh, lavender, frankincense, or coriander. For the best results, massage the salve into your stretch marks twice daily.

#64 Yogurt Cornmeal Face Scrub

To create a natural face scrub to clean your pores, combine ¼ cup cornmeal with ¼ cup plain yogurt in a small bowl. Mix well. In a small jar or bottle, combine 5 drops each of lavender, patchouli, and grapefruit and shake thoroughly. Pour the oils into the yogurt/cornmeal combo and stir all ingredients. Apply the mixture to your face, letting sit for 15-20 minutes, and then wash away. Any leftover scrub can be used for up to 3 days if covered and stored in the refrigerator.

#65 Nightly Face Moisturizer

Further improve your skin by applying this cleansing nightly face moisturizer. Simply combine 1 teaspoon carrier oil with 1 drop of lavender or frankincense oil. Mix well and apply to your face before you go to sleep. Rinse your face with water in the morning.

#66 Perfume

Essential oils can be used to personalize your own perfume. In a spray bottle, combine 1 ounce of high quality vodka with 25 drops of the essential oil(s) of your choice. Blend whatever combination appeals to you – lavender, geranium, sandalwood, and patchouli are lovely perfume scents. Before using, allow the perfume to age for 2 weeks. Then apply as usual, to your wrists and neck, or behind your ears and knees.

#67 Scented Lotion

You can also create a scented lotion. If used in combination with your perfume, your personalized scent will be even stronger and will last longer. Combine 25 drops of your personalized blend with 8 ounces of unscented lotion. Mix well and keep in an airtight container. For a sultry blend, combine 15 drops of geranium, 10 drops of myrrh, and 5 drops of ylang ylang with 8 ounces of unscented lotion.

#68 Sunscreen

If you fry like a lobster in the sun (even if you don't), you can produce your own 40 SPF sunscreen by combining in a small spray bottle, or other container, 40 drops of carrier oil with 20 drops each of carrot essential oil and myrrh. Apply as usual 15 minutes before sun exposure, and reapply every hour or so.

#69 Metabolism & Weight loss

Metabolism-Boosting Weight Loss Blend

By combining grapefruit, lemon, ginger, cinnamon, and peppermint you can personalize your own metabolism-boosting weight loss blend. Each of these essential oils benefits your body's metabolism and helps promote weight loss in its own way, which we'll detail below.

Grapefruit

Grapefruit essential oil promotes physical weight loss, along with addressing psychological issues that lead to binge-eating. Grapefruit oil targets cellulite and toning, combats overeating, and balances stress levels. It also harmonizes your mentality to diet, combating eating disorders and stimulating self-acceptance and healthy body image.

Lemon

Lemon essential oil boosts your body's energy levels, kills intestinal parasites, helps to detox the body, and mitigates digestive issues. Lemon oil can also aid in making health-conscious diet choices, as it improves judgement and body image.

Ginger

Ginger essential oil has long served in mitigating digestive issues as well. This oil can also be used as a tonic to stimulate and warm the body, boosting your energy. Often unhealthy diet and low energy are due to feelings of powerlessness and defeat. The psychological components of ginger essential oil provide increased empowerment, which promote psychological strength and a willingness to change.

Cinnamon

Cinnamon essential oil is an enhancer – it stimulates all other essential oils and aids in their cohesiveness. In and of itself, cinnamon oil helps circulation and digestion, produces better insulin levels, boosts the immune system, and detoxes the body, all of which aid the metabolism and promote weight loss. Psychologically, cinnamon essential oil promotes healthy body image, confidence and self-worth.

Peppermint

Peppermint essential oil aids digestion and lifts depression, by boosting motivation and optimism.

As you can see, each of these essential oils will assist both the mind and body in weight loss. Combine equal parts of each (20 drops will do) in a dark bottle, and shake well. Or you can test out different measurements of each oil to create your own personalized blend. Below are the recommended applications.

Balance Appetite

To maintain your appetite balance throughout the day, either inhale the oil blend directly from the bottle or apply 2-3 drops to each glass of water you drink.

Maintain Blood Sugar

Either apply 2-3 drops to each glass of water you drink or massage 3-4 drops into the soles of your feet twice a day.

Reduce Cellulite

Apply 1-2 drops topically to the affected area.

Promote Circulation

Apply 3-4 drops topically over the heart or other affected area every day.

Prevent Cravings

Inhale directly from the bottle or combine 1 ounce of water to 1 drop of the blend and drink.

Detox

Either apply 3-4 drops to each glass of water you drink or apply topically to the reflex points of your feet.

Alleviate Digestive Issues

Apply 1-2 drops topically over the abdomen or add 3-4 drops to a glass of water and drink as needed.

Boost Energy

Apply 1-2 drops to drinking water, rub topically into feet or diffuse.

Boost Metabolism

Rub topically into feet or apply 1-2 drops to each glass of water you drink

Chapter 4:
Essential Oils for Wellness

The medicinal uses of essential oils are unending. Those listed here in the *101 Uses of Essential Oils* eBook offer only a tiny glimpse into the medicinal benefits of essential oils. Check out our eBook *Essential Oils Survival Kit* for a more extensive and thorough list of the use of oils in maintaining your wellness.

#70 Insomnia

If you are prone to insomnia or you find you simply can't fall asleep every once in awhile, lavender essential oil is the answer. Combine 4-5 drops with 8 ounces of water in a spray bottle, and before bed each night, spritz your pillow. The lavender produces a soothing and calming effect, easing you off into sleep.

#71 Headaches

To address a mild headache, combine a teaspoon of carrier oil with 1 drop peppermint and 2 drops lavender. Using your fingers, massage the blend into your temples. The peppermint will ease your headache and the lavender will provide a calming effect.

#72 Congestion

If you have built-up congestion, bring water to a boil and fill a bowl with the steaming water. Mix in a few drops of eucalyptus or peppermint oil. With a towel or dishrag draped over your head, bend over the bowl and breathe deeply.

#73 PMS

To ease PMS, combine a teaspoon of carrier oil with 2-3 drops geranium or rosemary oil. Either add the combo to a hot bath or massage into the neck and shoulders. You can further ease menstrual cramps by combining 8 drops of carrier oil with 2 drops of basil, clary sage, or rosemary. Massage the blend into your lower abdomen and place a hot damp hand towel over your abdomen for 10-15 minutes.

#74 Toothache

¼ teaspoon of olive oil combined with 2 drops clove oil will offer temporary pain relief from a toothache. Dip a cotton ball in the blend and place it in your mouth alongside the affected tooth.

#75 Snoring

If you or your partner snores, an easy preventative remedy is to combine 3 drops of a carrier oil with 3 drops of thyme and apply to the bottoms of the feet before you go to sleep.

#76 Burns

Mild burns can be soothed and healed through the use of lavender essential oils. Simply apply a few drops topically to the burn. Be sure to test a small area of the burn before fully committing to the remedy.

#77 Blisters & Cold Sores

To soothe and heal blisters and cold sores, combine 1 drop of carrier oil with 1 drop helichrysum. Topically apply to the affected area 3 times daily or until the blister or cold sore disappears.

#78 Flu & Cold

An immune system booster will help your body combat any flu or cold symptoms. Whether you feel a cold or flu coming on or your illness is in full-swing, combine 1 drop of carrier oil and 1 drop of protective blend and apply to the soles of your feet twice a day.

#79 Nausea

If you are feeling nauseous, combine 4 drops of carrier oil with 1 drop nutmeg, patchouli, ginger, or peppermint. Mix well and apply topically on your abdomen and behind each ear 2-3 times every hour.

#80 First Degree Sunburn (no blisters)

To soothe a painful sunburn, combine 1 tablespoon of carrier oil with 2 drops Roman chamomile, rose, or lavender. Using a cotton ball, apply 1-3 drops topically to the sunburn. Inflammation will be reduced and the blend will promote healing. You can also run a cool bath and apply several drops of lavender oil to the bathwater, along with a nylon sock filled with oats. Both will soothe the skin and reduce inflammation.

Chapter 5:
Essential Oils for Travel

#81 Jet Lag Prevention & Reparation

DIY Jet Lag Prevention

Before you even set foot upon a plane, you can prevent jet lag using essential oils. How? Well, jet lag is influenced by dehydration, exhaustion and anxiety; so using essential oils, which help combat each, will allow you to maintain your electrolyte balance, sleep well, and reduce your stress.

Hydration

Apply a few drops of citrus or lemon essential oil to

your water to improve hydration and electrolyte balance before you travel.

Exhaustion

A lavender spritz on your pillow before you go to bed will help ease you into sleep, providing you the necessary rest you need before any big trip.

Anxiety

Relieving stress before any trip is key to reducing the effects of jet lag. Again, lavender essential oil is calming and can be inhaled or applied topically.

DIY Jet Lag Reparation

Adjust to the Time Zone

Once you arrive at your destination, it's important to adjust to the time zone you're in so that your jet lag doesn't affect you for an extended period of time. Citrus oils, like grapefruit, orange, lemon, spearmint and peppermint, are fantastic stimulants that will boost your energy, so you can make it through that first day and fall asleep at a normal hour in accordance with the time zone. Apply oil topically to your neck, head, and feet.

Take a Soothing Bath or Shower

Before you go to sleep, take a soothing bath to calm any stress from travel and help you sleep easier. Add some lavender or geranium essential oils to your Epsom salt (or regular table salt if you have none on hand) and throw these in your bath water. Lavender also eases muscle tension, so any muscle stress from travel will be relieved. Or, if you prefer a shower in the morning, plug the tub while you shower and place 2-3 drops peppermint, spruce, or eucalyptus essential oils to provide a morning energy boost.

#82 Travel Sanitizer

When you travel, you come into contact with lots of people, which means you come into contact with lots of germs. To produce an effective travel sanitizer, combine purified water with 8-10 drops of a protective blend in a spray bottle. Shake well and use as needed. You can kill germs everywhere on anything, from your hotel pillow cases and bed covers to public toilets and your hands after you've taken public transportation.

#83 Anxiety Calmer

Those who suffer from claustrophobia or have travel anxiety, particularly on planes, can either inhale a little chamomile or lavender essential oil, or rub it on the wrists before and during the feelings of anxiety.

#84 Immune Booster

As you travel and are bombarded with hundreds or thousands of people, your immune system will need to be strong to prevent sickness and to deal with germs. Create an immune booster by combining 4 drops of a carrier oil and 1 drop oregano. Massage this combo into the soles of your feet before, during, and after your travel.

#85 Motion Sickness

Peppermint essential oil will help those who suffer from motion sickness. Simply inhale the oil deeply or massage 2 drops into the abdomen.

Chapter 6:
Essential Oils for Gifting

#86 House-Warming

Give the gift of refreshing scent by creating your own wardrobe bags. Cut out squares of beautiful cotton material, apply 1-2 drops of lavender on the squares, then sew them up into bags to toss into drawers, closets, or wardrobes throughout your friend's new home.

#87 Bridal Shower Love Potion

Create a "love potion" set for the bride-to-be, including scented lotion and perfume. A fantastic perfume scent combines 1 drop rose, 4 drops cocoa, and 20 drops vanilla with 1-ounce high quality vodka. Shake well and pour into a vintage perfume bottle. For the lotion, combine

4 ounces carrier oil, 10 drops vanilla and 40 drops cocoa.

#88 Mother's Day

For Mother's Day, personalize a candle set with your mother's favorite scent. Fill a glass with 2 cups soy wax flakes. Cover with plastic wrap and in 10-second increments, melt the wax in the microwave, stirring each time with a wooden spoon. When the wax is completely melted, remove the plastic wrap and stir in 10 drops of the essential oil of your choice. Pour ½ inch of wax into a mason jar and stick a long wick (the height of the jar) into the wax. Continue pouring the remaining wax around the wick and hold it straight for 1-2 minutes, until the wax sets. If necessary, trim the wick to 1 inch above the wax and refrigerate for two hours or until the wax hardens.

#89 Gift for the Newly Pregnant

Your newly pregnant friend will thank you when you relieve her morning sickness and nausea with the gift of ginger, wild orange, peppermint, or lemon essential oil. Any of these oils can either be inhaled directly from the bottle or combined with carrier oil and rubbed on the belly. Use a high ratio of carrier to essential oil.

#90 Baby Shower

Provide your mother-in-waiting with a calming scent and diffuser so that baby and mother can sleep. Lavender is a very soothing scent that will calm a crying baby and ease relaxation.

#91 Winter Holiday Gift

During the winter holidays, spread Christmas cheer by sending scents to those you love. Vanilla, spruce, fir needle, cinnamon, pine, and clove will fill the homes of your friends and family with warmth from far away. Provide a diffuser or instruct your recipients to add several drops to a saucepan and simmer the water on the stove.

#92 Father's Day

If you have a hard-working father, then promote relief from stress this Father's Day by gifting him with a car diffuser and lavender oil. On the way to and from work, the oil will melt away anxiety and induce relaxation.

#93 Birthday Bath Salts

Everyone likes a nice relaxing bath, which is why pampering gifts – like these birthday bath salts – are a perfect way to personalize a scent for your friend or family member. To make bath salts, all you have to do is combine 1 cup baking soda with 1 cup Epsom salt and 20-30 drops of pure, or blended essential oil(s). Ylang ylang and lavender are always good for a calming bath. You can personalize the mason jar, or another bath salt container, and instruct your recipient to use ¼ cup each bath.

Chapter 7:
Essential Oils for Mood & Spirit

#94 Nerve/Anxiety Blend

If you suffer from nerves or anxiety, you can use a daily body lotion to calm both. Combine 9 drops carrier oil with 3 drops sweet marjoram or jasmine and apply every morning and evening or as needed throughout the day.

#95 Uplifting Blend

Although severe depression may be a chronic condition, the blues can be treated with essential oil. Roman chamomile, geranium, bergamot, sandalwood, and jasmine are all uplifting scents. Apply 1-3 drops topically or use as an inhalant, rubbing the drops in your palms, cupping them over your mouth and nose, and inhaling deeply. While applying, force your mind upon something that makes you happy.

#96 Mood Booster

Rose will alleviate stress, anxiety, and other depressive symptoms. Use as an inhalant, in a diffuser, or in your bath to boost your mood when you're feeling fatigued or stressed.

#97 Clarity

If you're in need of a clear mind, inhale 6-12 slow, deep huffs of frankincense before you go to sleep. Frankincense stimulates spiritual awakening, calms emotions, and produces clarity of mind.

#98 Anointing

Following the Christian Bible, myrtle, frankincense, cypress, or myrrh can be used to anoint someone in blessing or in prayer.

#99 Prayer

Another use of essential oil in prayer comes from none other than King David. In Psalm 51:10, the great king used hyssop as he prayed, "Create in me a clean heart oh God and renew a right spirit within me..." Combine 2-parts carrier oil to 1-part hyssop and apply to the neck and temples as you pray.

#100 Worship

When you're preparing to visit a place of worship, inhale or anoint yourself with cinnamon, or cassia essential oil, in line with the holy scriptures, Exodus 30:22-31.

#101 Meditation

If you practice yoga or meditation, inhale frankincense, orange, sandalwood, or rosemary essential oils to enhance your experience. These oils are known to create balance, harmony, and clarity.

Conclusion

As this book has demonstrated, the versatility, and beneficial qualities of essential oils is unparalleled. Synthetic man-made products cannot compare with the purity of nature and its countless uses when it comes to wellness, body, or home cleaning. These extracts from flowers, roots, leaves, berries, bark, roots, twigs, citrus peels, wood, and herbs are pure and effective in every sense of the word. Their powerful concentration and their derivation from nature's organic materials make them so.

However, it is important to note again that caution must be taken when using essential oils. When specified, always dilute your essential oils with a carrier oil. If you question whether or not the oil should be used "neat" or undiluted, then do a little research prior to use so that you know for sure that it's safe to use the oil directly. Also, always refer to your oil's instructions or other guides as to how many drops to apply. If using pure oil, in most cases, 4-5 drops topically on feet, palms or other body parts should be sufficient. If using for massage, dilute the oil around 30%.

If you have sensitive skin, always test in small doses before using topically over the entire affected area. Test on the inside of your upper arm and check for redness or irritation. If your skin does show some reaction, you can always dilute your oils with a carrier oil and try reapplying.

101 Uses of Essential Oils is dedicated to helping you find natural solutions to your wellness, your everyday household cleaning products, and your body, mind, and spirit. Give some of these DIY recipes, and remedies a shot, and you'll quickly be inspired to produce your own creative products with essential oils on your own terms.

DISCLAIMER AND/OR LEGAL NOTICES: Every effort has been made to accurately represent this book and it's potential. Results vary with every individual, and your results may or may not be different from those depicted. No promises, guarantees or warranties, whether stated or implied, have been made that you will produce any specific result from this book. Your efforts are individual and unique, and may vary from those shown. Your success depends on your efforts, background and motivation.

The material in this publication is provided for educational and informational purposes only and is not intended as medical advice. The information contained in this book should not be used to diagnose or treat any illness, metabolic disorder, disease or wellness problem. Always consult your physician or healthcare provider before beginning any nutrition or exercise program. Use of the programs, advice, and information contained in this book is at the sole choice and risk of the reader.